She Time

The Woman's Guide to a Keen Mind and Thin Body

By Tommy Highway

I would like to start off by introducing myself. My name is Tommy and I am a fitness instructor. I began my career many years ago after losing nearly 80 pounds. The experience was life altering to say the least. It inspired me to become a fitness instructor and to help others change their lives for the better. Not long into my career, I discovered something about human nature; women tend to want to improve themselves more so than men. Women also tend to care a great deal more about their health, fitness, and personal appearance. So I began to specialize in the female form. I reviewed countless books and media on the subject of female anatomy, metabolism, and even changes brought on by menopause. What were the best types of exercises, the best foods, even down to the best time of day for a woman to have meals? What I really couldn't find were many well written publications that discussed the real reasons that a woman would gain weight. What was her mindset, what were her general dietary habits, and what were effective support methods? Yes, there was a great deal of information out there, but I could find nothing that really tied it all together so I formulated my own approach. To my surprise frankly, my methods were not only getting results, they were getting fabulous results. I decided to write this book to offer my methods to all of the wonderful women out there who are ready to get not only physically fit, but also mentally fit. You see, I realized that it is impossible to have one without the other. After all, our mothers, our daughters, our wives, and our partners are the most important people in our lives.

Any woman's journey into physical fitness must include four components: proper exercise, proper diet, a proper support system, and MOST importantly, a proper mindset. Think of your journey in terms of a well-oiled machine. The machine runs well until a component breaks down. When this happens the machine breaks down. We are going to discuss these four components in detail in the pages that follow. Before we go any further there is something that you must know. You are about to start a journey that will not only change your body, it will also change many aspects of your life in a very positive way. Our goal here is to change what I call your level of thinking and being. I know what you are probably thinking right now, I am not going to ask you to sit in a drum circle, chant, or even sing folk songs. Simply put, we are going to change your personal negatives into positives. We are going to change the way that you look at the most important person in your life and that person is you. In working with women, I have come to understand and appreciate your daily stresses. After all, you may have a career, a family to care for, a needy partner, and this puts a great deal of pressure on you. The important thing to understand here is that you MUST take some She time. This may seem difficult at first; however, as you move forward it will get easier and you will be much happier I promise! The important thing to remember here is not that you can do this, but that you WILL do this.

Whether you are looking for a complete body transformation or just need a tune up, She time can and will work for you. Whatever the reasons are that you have gained weight be it medical, social, interpersonal, childbirth, or any other reason, just know that I have personally witnessed women move mountains and I know that you will too. You are the author of the book of your life and every day you get to write another page. You are the director of your own movie and it's time for the next scene. The good news is that you get to decide how the storyline plays out. Let's get started writing your new story today.

Dedicated to Karen Lees. Mother to many, friend to all

Contents

Chapter 1

The She Time Mind

The most important part of any body transformation is the mind. It doesn't matter whether you are male or female, young or old, or where you are from. Your attitude, mood, and personal faith are directly responsible for your success or failure. Your fitness journey both begins and ends in the mind. Now let's take a look at that word "failure". This is not a word that you will see a great deal of in this book. You see both your success and failure have one thing in common YOU. Everyone's life has ups and downs. The problem is that in many cases the "downs" tend to affect our attitude much more than the "ups" and the reason for this is that unfortunately, we tend to allow our "downs" to linger and our "ups" to be short-lived. You must understand that science has proven that a positive thought is many times more powerful than a negative thought. The good news is that you can control this. When our life faces adversity, it is very important to realize that these situations are temporary. You may have relationship issues, financial issues, career issues, or family issues. It is important to realize that these issues can and will be corrected through proper thinking. That's right, I said proper thinking. It is extremely important to replace the feeling of being trapped with the feeling of being free. This is accomplished by being aware of your current thoughts. When you are experiencing thoughts of feeling trapped, it is very easy to recognize and change them. Whenever you begin to feel stressed or overwhelmed it's time to make some She Time. Try putting on some music, think of happy memories, pull out a photo album, drop a comedy into the DVD player. These are just some of the easy ways that you can begin to change your thought process. Laughter really is the best medicine so give it a try.

It is time to begin our first exercise. I would like for you to put this book down and go find a large mirror. Take a look at yourself and I mean really look deeply. Go ahead and spend some time staring at your image. It is important to focus on yourself as a whole and not to be drawn to any one particular feature or perceived imperfections. I would like for you to take a deep breath and say the following words, "I am a beautiful woman". Say it out loud, repeat it, and don't worry nobody is watching. It is very important for you to believe your own words because it happens to be the truth. Whether you are a size 0 or size 44, you are already a work of art. As a great artist once so eloquently put it "Every block of stone has a statue inside it and it is the task of the sculptor to discover it." - Michelangelo. Ladies, you are about to become the artist.

It is very important to keep in mind that all that you can do is to improve on your own personal perfection. This level of positive thinking is absolutely imperative for success in anything that we do in life. The catch is that you, and only you, can improve yourself. You are the painter of your own life canvas. You can only get better. This may be a difficult concept to grasp at first as every woman has things about her body that they well, just don't care for. I don't want you to focus on your self-perceived imperfections. That is a major step in the wrong direction. It is very important for you to focus not so much on who you are at the moment, but the person that you WILL become. Sure, I could tell you that there are many people that count on you to be mentally and physically healthy, and I would be correct. Chances are that if you are reading this book then you may be a mother, a wife, a sister, a daughter, and those are wonderful titles to own. In fact, the more love that you have surrounding you the better. As wonderful as it is to be part of a relationship and a family the truth is that this journey is only about you, and you must undertake it only for YOU. You must take She Time.

Now let's discuss one of your mind's most important needs. I call it "She" Time. She Time is the time that you set aside each day that is only for you. I have found that 20-30 minutes each day is the perfect amount of time for our mental exercises. You need 30 minutes for yourself every day and with all that you do, you deserve 30 minutes a day of She Time. I understand that circumstances in your life may be hectic and you may not feel that you have enough time to accomplish everything that you need to do in a day however, you can always find that crucial 30 minutes. Don't worry, the universe will not grind to a halt and your loving family will understand. I just can't stress enough the importance of your mind and thought process. Your positive thoughts and mood are so important for success. They are crucial to your personal success.

Now that we have established our She time let's talk about the importance of having and maintaining a positive mood. Have you ever noticed that if something goes wrong in the morning that the rest of the day tends to go badly? Think about it, you slip in the shower, you stub your toe, perhaps the alarm didn't go off. It could be any negative experience and you face nothing but drama for the rest of the day. Why? Because whatever negative event that started your day off poorly is now dominating your thoughts, and your thoughts are creating negative emotions and those negative emotions are creating your bad mood which in turn, creates more negative thoughts and... you end up in a vicious cycle with only one loser YOU. The key is to recognize the negative event and stop it in its tracks.

Let's try something, the next time that you wake up and experience a negative event STOP. It's important for you to realize that whatever just happened is probably not the end of the world. Take a few minutes to breathe deep and relax. Put on your favorite song, hug someone, pet the cat, these are just some examples of ways to bring yourself back into a positive mindset. Ladies, a positive mindset is so important that it is nearly impossible to put into words. Think of it this way, we have all had an unfortunate run-in with an unpleasant person right? The next time this happens take a really good look at that person. I'll bet that they look older than they actually are. I'll bet that most of them aren't very healthy or for that matter, pleasant in appearance.
They look this way because frankly, they have allowed negative thoughts and emotions to literally become toxic within their own bodies as well as their personal reality. Unfortunately, these unpleasant few have never realized that with a basic change of mindset, they could be as happy and healthy as you are going to be.

Another key to any transformation is visualization. Ladies you need to declare within your own mind exactly what you want to accomplish. Not hope, not wish, but you need to know deep down what it is that you want. You must have no doubt as to exactly what you are about to accomplish. You need not worry about the how, we will get to that. It is important to hold those thoughts in your mind and refer to them often. A wonderful way of establishing exactly what it is that you want is to simply grab a pen and a notebook. Write those desires down and literally declare what you want. Make this your predominant thought. Slip that notebook into your purse and refer to it often. I have found that keeping my notebook on my nightstand is an enormous help. When I wake up in the morning the first thing I do is look at my list. When you walk over and look in that mirror, I want you to see a fit person looking back at you. I want you to see a happy and prosperous person looking back at you. I want you to see yourself exactly the way that you want to look and more importantly, I want you to feel the way that you want to feel. The power of visualization can be such a powerful experience and is certainly a wonderful motivational tool. Lay back, close your eyes and think about the perfect scene. It could be on a beautiful island, maybe a cruise; just whatever you feel would be the perfect experience. Now place yourself in the scene. I'm not talking about the past you, I'm not talking about the current you; I'm speaking of the future you. See yourself in a beautiful evening gown, mingle with people. It's all about YOU. It is really important to take a few minutes each day for this exercise. This may seem unrealistic and even silly at first; however this can be one of the most powerful motivational tools in your personal arsenal. Remember that visualization is a step forward, and a step forward is always a step in the right direction. It is very important to remember that your thoughts really do make your own reality whether you realize it or not. I understand that this concept, at first glance, almost feels like you are lying to yourself. To that I would dust off an oldie saying that it isn't a lie, if you believe it.

When you imagine that your body is transforming, you will be amazed that it actually begins to happen. The key is to believe that you are improving within your own mind. Remember that thoughts tend to become reality whether they are positive or negative. Think about it, throughout human history, who were the most successful people? They were the positive thinkers. They were people who simply had the "Big Picture" mindset. Once you master your mind and mood, you will become unstoppable. Just remember that you can't be it until you think it.

Now let's take some She Time and do a basic 5 minute exercise. You will need to go someplace that is quiet with no interruptions. Now let's sit in a comfortable position and completely relax your body. Honestly, you will need to get comfy for this. Now close your eyes and breathe deeply. Clear your mind of any thoughts and think of a ripe lemon. Rotate the lemon in your mind and look at the detail of the skin. Look at the bright yellow color. When other thoughts come into your mind remember that this is normal and natural; however you must recognize this and focus right back on the lemon. This is a short exercise that basically trains your mind to focus on one subject and block everything else out. At first, you might find it difficult to focus on the lemon and keep other thoughts at bay; however as you repeat this exercise you will find it much easier to concentrate. The more time you spend on this exercise you will notice that you will be able to focus on the lemon for longer periods of time. This will begin to make you happier and more focused almost immediately. Keeping the mind focused is the key.

The power of the mind cannot be overstated. It is the source of either your success or failure; however the good news is that you have the power to harness and control your own thoughts. If you feel "bad" most of the time, you will tend to feel that way more and more often. You literally become not just the product of, but also the source of negative energy. Science has proven long ago that everything and everyone is made up of energy. The important thing to realize is that energy that is in a negative state tends to affect and corrupt positive energy. In other words, when you are in a negative state of mind or mood, the other people, places, and things around you are likely to be effected in a negative way.

To break this down a bit further and at the risk of sounding cliché, misery loves company. You may have issues in your life that may feel hopeless. Perhaps you are having relationship, family, or financial difficulties. No matter what your personal issues are, the only way to begin to change your life is to start on an interpersonal level. You need to start feeling good about you. It is important that you don't create your own depression. Always remember that you are the solution not the problem. You must understand and believe that you can conquer any problem that comes your way. It is also important to be grateful for the things you already have. Everyone has something that they are proud of. Maybe it's your family, your career, perhaps even the clothes that you wear. The important thing is to recognize what you are grateful for, proud of, and focus on the feelings and emotions that you receive by thinking of them.

The truth is gratitude tends to bring about more reasons to feel grateful. You may not have the perfect life; however there is always something that you are grateful for. Capture those images and emotions and hold them in your mind. Go ahead and break out your notebook. On the page opposite your desires list, I want you to create a list of the things that you are grateful for. The more that you focus on the positive aspects of your life, the more positive aspects you will have to focus on, and that is the promise of the universe.

Just remember, positive thoughts are many times more powerful than negative thoughts. I am not suggesting that you monitor all of your thoughts as that would be impossible and somewhat maddening. The trick is in how you deal with negative thoughts and circumstances as they occur. You must learn to replace negative thoughts with positive thoughts. This may seem like a lot of work at first; however as you make these changes it will become easier and commonplace within your own mind. This is the point at which your mindset begins to naturally evolve into positive territory. Remember, once you own your thoughts, you can own anything that you wish for. You become the genie of the lamp.

Now let's talk about weight gain and how it affects the way you feel. Again, it is important to realize that the weight gain is not about who you are. It's about who you were. Depression is one of the leading causes of weight gain. You may have a negative opinion of yourself because you don't look the same as you did in high school. Perhaps you haven't lost the baby weight. Whatever the reason, it is important to replace those negative feelings with positive feelings in order to move forward. Your spouse or partner can be either an asset or a liability as their opinion of you is obviously important. The truth is that most partners tend to handle their partner's weight gain poorly. Many of them have yet to realize that complaining is only creating more reason to complain. They really have no idea that being negative toward you is only making matters worse. After all, this is your partner, and we look to our partners for many of our strengths and when our partner is unsupportive then they become almost the enemy of your positive thoughts. Partners tend not to realize that words can cut deeply into a woman's psyche and cause long-term damage not only to her emotions, but to the overall relationship. This emotional damage is cumulative. These, along with all of the other daily stresses that are unique to women, make for a perfect storm of negative attitude and emotion.

I have personally witnessed so many partners make these mistakes that I am actually considering writing a chapter in the back of this book just for them. Again, when dealing with this kind of negativity it is absolutely imperative to keep your mind and thoughts in a positive state. When presented with someone else's negative thoughts and-or emotions it is ok to walk away and regroup, while holding the thoughts of gratitude and freedom in your mind. This may be difficult at first; however, it will get easier as you move forward. I am certainly not suggesting that you become selfish or neglect anyone; however it is important to remember that this journey is about you. This is about She Time. Your thoughts really do need to be predominantly about you at this time.

Another wonderful tool for keeping yourself positive and focused is most likely already in your possession. If you own a marker, paper, and some tape, then you already have one of the best motivational tools that I have ever used. I'm talking about the ability to create signs for yourself and strategically place them about your home. Let's be honest, as fallible human beings we have a tendency to allow our good intentions to fade away as time goes on. With everything that we have on our daily plate it is very easy to procrastinate and put things off for a better time. It is important to remember that standing still is really no different than a step backward. A step backward is always a step in the wrong direction. This is why we must constantly remind ourselves of our purpose which is to improve both the mind and the body.

Let's try another exercise. Lay out five sheets of paper on a table. Close your eyes and breathe deeply while thinking about all of the things that you are about to accomplish. Remember that it is extremely important for your thoughts to be both positive and forward. Think of what you are about to accomplish and feel good about it. It doesn't matter whether or not you are where you want to be yet; the most important thing to remember is that you need to feel like you are already there. Believe it. Believe it. Believe it. You are in the creative process. You are literally changing your own reality. Give yourself some time with this and remember that visualization is not a race.

The practice of visualization takes time to learn. Think of it as a brick building and you build it brick by brick. After you feel calm and comfortable, I want you to open your eyes. Think of five inspirational words or short sayings. Feel free to congratulate yourself for taking this next step because it is huge. Now let's break out the marker and write those thoughts down on the paper before you. These should be interpersonal, inspirational words and thoughts that are unique to your own desires. Remind yourself of what you really want. Hold those thoughts in your mind and most importantly, believe that they have already happened in your heart of hearts.

Think of your signs as focal points. They are signposts of what lies just ahead. Road signs to guide you through the journey. Now that we have created our signs let's place them in locations in your home where you spend most of your time. When you feel stressed, depressed, angry, or any other negative emotion, simply find one of your signs and focus. Take a minute to breathe deeply and think of the lemon. It is important to concentrate on the positive thought that you have created on that sign. This is She Time. This really will help your mindset stay in positive territory. Although your signs are personal thoughts there is one sign in particular that is standard and universally works for everyone.

That is a simple sign that is placed on the refrigerator and pantry. This sign should be written by your own hand to ask yourself one simple question, do I want this? When you have the urge to snack, look at your sign, close your eyes and go to that party, eat dinner at the Captain's table, put on that gown. Work it girl. Go where you really want to be in your mind. Again ladies, remember that when you visualize you materialize. Let that positive emotion flow through your mind and simply walk away from that temptation. During my own personal transformation one of the things that made me particularly proud was a simple trip to the supermarket. Once I finally put all of the pieces together, my mind, my diet, my exercise program, I could actually walk up to the bakery counter and have the willpower to simply smile and tell the baker that I'm just looking. That in itself was one of the most empowering moments of my life as I am a hopeless chocoholic...

Chapter 2

The She Time Diet

efore beginning any diet or exercise program it is extremely important to consult your physician. Ladies, it is just a smart thing to do. Now that we have started to change your thought process, let's talk about your diet. What you put into your body really does matter. I want you to remember something very important, if you don't put it into your mouth, then it can't go to your belly, legs, and rear. Keep in mind that your body does not create fat out of thin air. It is simply reacting to the foods that you are feeding it. I understand that in today's society it is very easy to get busy and eat the most convenient source of food. You guessed it; I'm talking about through the window, in the box, speak into the clown's head fast food. Have you ever taken the time to check the fat and calorie content of some of the more popular options out there? In some cases one sandwich can be as many as 650 calories, and the average fast food meal is a whopping 900 calories. Let's not forget all of the fat and additives that are being injected into your system. Eating these kinds of foods may be convenient and they might even seem cheap; however I can promise that you are getting exactly what you are paying for. Take a look at the people you know that consume vast quantities of fast food. Bet that they look it right? Let me ask you to ponder another question, have you ever eaten fast food and felt good afterward?

Now let's talk about these super, wonderful, miracle diets that get so much attention every year or so. I have personally tried many of the "fad" diets out there and have found many of them to be just another smoke and mirror opportunity to sell a book, video, or box of "natural" food delivered to your door. Fad diets come and go for one simple reason; every woman's body is different. Simply put, what may be right for Karen's body may not work for Amanda. I have found it helpful to teach my clients to view their body as a combination lock. You see every woman's body has its own individual combination and when you discover the correct combination you will unlock your body's potential and literally become its master. Now, I'm obviously not speaking of a set of numbers, I am speaking of the right foods, exercise, and mindset. It really is a formula. Many of my clients have been ladies who tend to prefer to eat out because of one small issue, they cannot cook. What you need to understand about finding your body combination is to keep it very simple. If you own basic cookware and have a heat source then you are all set. By keeping it simple, I'm speaking of meals that are quick and easy to prepare. Think chicken stir fry, think lean pork, think fish, you will be amazed at the filling meals that you can make with just some vegetables, cheese, a few spices, and a meat. In fact, I am going to provide you with a basic formula in the pages that follow.

I am certainly not writing this to endorse any one particular product; however I am a HUGE fan of a certain former boxer's grill that is on the market. I will refer to it as the "Boxer" grill here in the book. This is an absolutely amazing way to cook healthy while keeping it clean and simple. The Boxer grill comes in many different sizes from a single portion to a family size meal. Best of all, you can prepare a meat and vegetable meal very quickly, and at virtually the same time, without creating a mess. It's even more efficient than turning on your range so you can feel green about it. The Boxer grill is so infinitely versatile that I am considering writing a cookbook with it specifically in mind. These units are relatively inexpensive and the single serving models are downright cheap.

Keeping your diet basic is certainly the way to go for numerous reasons. Remember that simple does not mean boring. The key factor is that you want to know everything that is going into your body. At first glance this thought may seem unrealistic; however once you get your meal routine down and a little knowledge, you will find that daily meal preparation will become not only easy, but also very personally fulfilling. You are about to become creator of your own diet and your own success. You have read this far into this book because you have dedicated yourself to living a better quality of life. You want to be healthy and beautiful and you will absolutely achieve that goal. This journey starts with the mind, travels through the body, and ends with your personal happiness. There are a few stops along the way and the kitchen is a very important part that.

The simple truth is that in most cases weight gain is simply the result of your mind and body being out of alignment. This tends to cause depression and stress, and food becomes the medicine to treat the symptoms of that. I'm sure that you have all heard the term "comfort food" right? Unfortunately, it is a lie that we tell ourselves over and over. Think of it this way, you get depressed so you eat something. After eating whatever it was, you get depressed because you have eaten it, which in turn leads to more thoughts of depression and a vicious cycle that seems never ending. This unfortunately, is why many women simply lose hope. They give into these negative emotions and therefore they imprison themselves instead of empowering themselves. They are literally creating a reality in which they become their own jailer. Ladies, this really is a self-inflicted wound and is happening simply because you have never had the right combination to unlock your body's potential. It is important not to blame yourself. Again, the weight isn't about who you are, it's about who you were. You have simply never been presented with this knowledge and way of thinking. Fat is, in the most basic terms, stored energy.

Think of it as the ghost of dinner's past. Ladies, we are about to exorcise the demons. You are about to turn that stored energy into positive energy. Think of it this way, all your life you have been putting into your body whatever you want, and neglecting what your body actually needs. You have been doing this not because you haven't had the proper foods available, or were unable to hear your body's song, you simply couldn't understand the melody. This is where all of our exercises from the previous chapter begin to provide the light for the path forward. The good news is that a simple change in diet can do amazing things for not only your body, but also your emotional state. This begins to happen almost immediately. A proper diet will promote alignment and provide a very positive almost never ending source of energy and sense of well-being. This sense of well-being is what makes this entire process work. This is what makes your life work. This is what brings you joy. Most importantly, this is what makes your thoughts and desires manifest into reality. Your body responds to the food that you put into it second only to your thoughts. If you eat unhealthy foods then you will be much more likely to be in a bad mood because simply put, your body is not working correctly. You are not in alignment. A change in your diet can also aid in menstrual cycle regulation and be of great importance during the entire menopausal process. A proper diet will also help prevent and reverse a range of diseases that are unique to women.

I would like to discuss one of the most preventable, yet debilitating diseases unique to women that I have ever encountered. I am speaking of Osteoporosis. According to most studies, 1 out of 2 women will experience an Osteoporosis related fracture in her lifetime. Consider Grandmother's hump. This condition is very common in elderly women. In most cases, this is simply the result of a lifetime diet that lacked one of the world's most common minerals. I am speaking of calcium. Several years ago I worked at a gym and met a lady in her mid-40's. Let's call her Angie.

This woman was in very good condition and by all accounts appeared to be aging very well. Angie began taking my group fitness classes and instantly fell in love with the power of group fitness. She would attend several classes per week and was losing a great deal of weight. Her muscles were firming and she appeared to be the picture of health. Suddenly, and without warning, Angie had an accident in class and broke her leg. Although serious injuries in fitness classes are extremely rare, they are not unheard of. Angie naturally assumed that she had simply taken a bad step and that it could have happened to anyone. After several weeks in a leg cast Angie was given a clean bill of health and she returned to her favorite group fitness class. Though it wasn't easy to get back into peak condition, Angie was very determined, so she fought through it and pressed on.

Just a few short weeks later, Angie was getting out of her car in a downpour when suddenly she felt an excruciating pain in her left ankle. Although she was in extreme pain, Angie was able to pivot back into the car and drive herself to a nearby hospital. Her diagnosis was a severely broken ankle. How could this be she thought? How could a simple everyday action like getting out of a car break a bone she thought? Angie decided to make an appointment to visit her family doctor. Her doctor was naturally concerned about her recent injuries so she ordered a series of tests including a bone density test. Angie's doctor discovered something terrible. Her diagnosis was advanced Osteoporosis. A lifetime diet lacking in basic minerals had made her bones so weak that they had become dangerously brittle. Angie's doctor had no choice but to immediately restrict her physical activities as any stress on her body could be dangerous. She was even warned that basic sexual activity could be problematic.

Obviously Angie was absolutely devastated at the diagnosis and immediately began several medications and forms of therapy. The major problem with Osteoporosis is that it is a condition that takes years or even decades to manifest. Treatment options are limited and no cure exists. Osteoporosis is one of the reasons that I am such a big believer in dairy products, or for those of you who are lactose intolerant, a dairy substitute such as soy or almond milk. Your body needs calcium and if you feed it properly you will be much happier and healthier in your golden years. We are all aware of how dangerous a broken bone can be to the elderly. Ladies, do yourself a huge favor and get a bone density test as soon as possible. If caught early, there are treatment options available including medications that require only one dose per month. Ladies it is very important to maintain regular visits with your doctor.

Please don't forget about your mammograms. There are two other tests that are important for every woman: You should also consider an iron and cholesterol test. This is basic information that everyone should know about themselves. The good news is that there is a simple way of obtaining these tests and it is even free of charge. Simply make a blood donation with the American Red Cross. They will run both of these tests on the same visit and have the results ready in a very short time. This is another one of those wonderful scenarios where everyone involved wins.

Many foods have been known for their healing and spiritual properties by many cultures over the last few thousand years. In fact, you might be hard pressed to find a fruit, vegetable, or even a tree on this planet that hasn't been harvested and used medicinally by humans. Alchemists in the Dark Ages believed certain herbs exhibited magical properties. Even today a large part of the pharmaceutical industry revolves around testing plants and fungi in hopes of creating the next miracle treatment or cure for disease. After all, penicillin was discovered growing on fruit.

The truth is that as humans were testing every food that we could find for medicinal properties throughout our history, we were fortunate enough to have found a great many more hits than misses. We discover, or rediscover superfoods all the time. One of the most important elements of a weight loss diet happens to be one of these ancient superfoods. It is even cheap and easy to find. I am speaking of green tea. It has been said that green tea was discovered in the Yunnan Province of China sometime before 1000 BC. Throughout history green tea has been known to promote everything from fertility to spiritual enlightenment. One thing that most doctors and scientists agree on today is that green tea is a powerful antioxidant and is known to promote a higher metabolic rate. One thing that I can tell you from personal experience is that green tea is simply an incredible weight loss tool. Its importance in speeding up your metabolism simply cannot be overstated. We will talk more about metabolism later. Your local supermarket will have several brands to choose from. Try to avoid the bottled green tea and brew your own. If you have been cleared by your doctor for caffeine use, then I suggest steering away from the decaf. I have had much better results from the caffeinated variety. The only down-side to green tea is the taste. Although some brands do taste better than others, if you find it unpalatable then feel free to sweeten it with lemon or a touch of honey. As for the dosage, I have had great results with one cup in the morning, one at lunch, and one mid-afternoon. If the caffeine is keeping you awake at night or you are having any physical issues then try adjusting the amount consumed or the times. Green tea is providing you with two wonderful benefits. It is not only speeding up your metabolism, it is also cleansing your body of toxins that have been building up over time. It really is a win-win.

Another miracle of the modern era may just be one of the most body friendly inventions of the last several decades. I am speaking of the juicer. I am a firm believer that every healthy body should own a juicer. Every living person should be issued one of these things. Several years ago a friend introduced me to juicing and I became hooked almost immediately. He loaded the juicer with several different varieties of fruits and vegetables and produced a concoction that was honestly not very appealing to the eye. This wonderful mixture of raw vitamins, minerals, and macronutrients certainly didn't taste like fruit punch for that matter. However within just a few minutes of ingesting my first glass of this juice, I felt what can only be described as a power surge. It was as if a great fire had been lit from within my body. I was extremely focused and overflowing with energy. I did some research on juicing and decided that I was bold enough to take on a seven day juice only diet commonly known as a juice fast, as a personal challenge.

I began my juice fast on a Monday having created my first pitcher of juice the night before. I had basically come up with a recipe consisting of apples, cucumbers, red cabbage, kale, and carrots. I would have an 8oz glass of juice at about 250 calories every 4 hours so about four glasses a day. Honestly, the first 3 days were not pleasant. The body will take some time to adjust to a total liquid diet. After my body adjusted I became completely energized to the point at which I was losing sleep. Then it occurred to me that I wasn't losing sleep, I just didn't require as much. I had not felt this kind of an energy rush since my teenage years and I was enjoying it. After about the 4th day I could really tell the difference in the fit of my clothing. Suddenly my pants were loose around my waist. I did notice something else, and there is no elegant way to put this so here goes... my body was expelling things that I may have been carrying around in my system for a long while possibly even years. At the end of my fast I had lost 13 pounds and felt completely refreshed inside and out. Another benefit that I noticed was that my skin, nails, and hair had never been in better shape. A juice fast is not for everyone and I do not endorse the process to be honest. I was amazed at how the years and sun damage on my skin had seemingly melted away. I was glowing..... and I'm a guy.

Unfortunately one of the most common issues with significant weight loss is the excess skin afterward. This can be an issue depending on many factors such as body mass, age, amount of weight lost, etc. A diet that is high in natural vitamin C as well as other natural vitamins and minerals can help your body shrink much of this excess tissue naturally as you lose weight making it less of an issue and much more manageable. Ladies, the juicer can be your best friend during the weight loss process. When it comes to purchasing a juicer, money really does matter. Although some less expensive models will do the job, remember that this is definitely the kind of purchase where you get what you pay for. Be prepared to spend around $100. As for juice recipes, there are many wonderful books, videos, and apps available to assist you. Feel free to experiment with all kinds of fruit and vegetable combinations. Don't worry, you will get used to the taste and you can always sweeten up your juice by adding more apples, carrots, and sweeter fruits like grapes. You will be amazed at what 2-3 daily glasses of natural, unpasteurized juice will do for your body. You can always tell if a person is a regular juicer as they typically have great skin and a natural glow about them. Think about this, when was the last time that you sat down and consumed 4 carrots, a cucumber, 2 apples, and an orange in one sitting? The juicer makes this level of nutrition easy and available to anyone with the right knowledge.

Over the years recommended diet practices have changed so many times that it is difficult to keep up with the latest information. There has been, and always will be a great debate between doctors, scientists, and nutritionists about exactly what the body requires. This debate has at times added more confusion than useful information to an already complex topic. Studies tend to compete and contradict each other much more than the average person can fathom. The American FDA has recommended a daily caloric intake of 2000–2500 for the average person. I personally believe that this number is grossly exaggerated. If I were to consume 2000 calories per day I would be about 60 pounds overweight. I know this because I have personally been there, eating by those rules. I have also never known anyone to actually lose weight consuming daily calories that were even close to those numbers. In my personal experience, the magic number to strive for is around 1300 calories per day. This number may be "hard to swallow" on first thought because it just does not sound like very much food right?

Close your eyes and use your new power of visualization to imagine tomorrow's meal:

Monday

Breakfast	Lunch	Dinner
1 pkg flavored oatmeal 1 8oz glass of juice 1 cup green tea	½ Chicken Mozzarella 1 cup mixed vegetable 1 sugar free pudding pop 8oz. milk or substitute 1 glass of juice 1 cup green tea	½ Chicken Mozzarella 1 cup mixed vegetable 1 slice of Texas toast 8oz milk or substitute 2 cups chocolate mousse

Looks good doesn't it? This is just an example of a daily meal plan. You may be surprised to know that this entire meal is about 1000 calories. Ladies, this really is a lot of food for a day. This meal is extremely filling and still has everything that your body needs to be healthy and efficient.

With a name like Chicken Mozzarella, this meal may seem intimidating to prepare; however it really is quite easy when done on the Boxer grill. If you happen to be at least a semi-conscious shopper then the approximate cost of this meal is around $8.00. That is just $8.00 per day. This meal is quick, delicious, filling, provides everything you need, and it is also less expensive than many fast food options.

Let's break this meal down into its basic ingredients:

Ingredient	Calories
1 packet of instant oatmeal (any flavor)	150
16oz of fresh made green juice (2 servings)	175
10oz boneless, skinless chicken breast	150
16oz of fat free milk or substitute	180
1 slice mozzarella cheese	90
½ cup of your favorite spaghetti sauce	45
1 slice Texas toast	140
2 sugar free pudding pops	70

Entree preparation is easy. Simply lay the slightly flattened chicken breast on the Boxer grill and add your favorite spices. After the chicken has been properly cooked remove from the grill and place it on a microwave safe dish. Place a slice of mozzarella on the chicken and pour your spaghetti sauce over it. Place the dish in the microwave for about 30 seconds to heat the sauce and finish melting the cheese. While your grill is still warm place your garlic toast on the Boxer grill for a few minutes. Preparation times will vary; however once you get your dining routine down you can actually prepare an entire daily meal in about 20 minutes. This meal has been outlined to provide you with a basic daily dietary formula.

This formula is high in vitamins and protein and low in fats and carbs. I am personally a big believer in low carbs versus no carbs. Carbohydrates are not necessarily the enemy so long as they are consumed in strict moderation. You will also want to avoid foods like white rice and products like pasta and most breads as these foods basically turn to sugars within the body. You may be thinking to yourself that the same meal for lunch and dinner might get boring after a while and you would be correct. The key to this method is to have a different dish for each meal.

Let's say you prepare Chicken Mozzarella for dinner on Monday night. You will want to divide the meal into two equal portions. The idea is to eat one portion for dinner and place the other portion in a covered dish in the refrigerator. The second portion will be lunch for Tuesday. Then on Tuesday evening you prepare a different meal and repeat the process. Half is for dinner, half is for lunch the next day. You will be amazed at how well this process will work for you. Feel free to change things up using the same basic formula. Think lean pork with brown rice, think fish, think just about any lean meat with a vegetable. One very important thing to remember is that spices weigh nothing. Every meal that you create is a meal to be proud of. You have already seen the light at the end of the tunnel and your meals are the vehicle fuel in which to get you to that light. Be creative with this, meal creation is a fun experience. Experiment and remember that meal creation should never be a chore within your mind. Feel joy in the fact that you are actually creating your own success. You are literally watching it happen with each bite at the end of your fork. It is certainly helpful to plan on having your meals at roughly the same time of day and evening. I realize that this may not always be possible; however, your body will tend to respond better if you stick to a routine. You will also want to avoid eating your meals in the late evening whenever possible. I have always used the no later than 3 hours before bedtime rule. Always remember that meal time is She Time. Feel free to congratulate yourself for completing this step in the process. You have just taken another major step in the right direction.

One of the things that we as humans have simply lost in the modern age is respect for our food. Think about it, food is everywhere. Our ancestors were forced to hunt down and kill their own food when available, while today most of us can jump in our car and be at the nearest supermarket in minutes. It has almost become too easy. So as a result of ease and abundance, we tend to overconsume and basically take our food for granted. We shovel it in because we know that there is plenty more where that came from. Overconsumption leads to the creation of fat. If you consume more calories than you burn in a daily period then your body will store those calories as fat which is Human Physiology 101.

So now that you have personally created a wonderful, healthy meal it is time for our next exercise. This can be done at lunch or dinner; however it would be best if you were alone without distraction. This is one of those She Time moments that we discussed earlier. You will need to lay out the wonderful meal that you just created on a table before you. Feel good about this meal. You really should feel very accomplished at this moment. Candlelight makes everything taste better so feel free to fire one up.

Now take your first bite and close your eyes. Enjoy the taste on your tongue. Enjoy the sensation of all of the ingredients happily mixing together in your mouth.

Roll your tongue around and enjoy the texture of your creation. You want to chew very slowly and truly enjoy the experience of your food.

You are literally eating your success and making it a part of you. Now let your mind go to that special place. Put on that gown, go to that party. It's all about you. This is your She Time. Use the power of visualization to equate the look and taste of your food to positive thoughts and emotions. When you learn to truly appreciate and respect your meal and feel gratitude for the entire process of its creation, then you have truly found the path to success. All that is left for you to do is to continue to move forward so enjoy the ride.

One of the biggest challenges during my journey was my sweet tooth. My particular vice of choice is chocolate. I will admit that it was the most difficult thing to give up. Then I realized that I didn't have to. I discovered the wonders of sugar free instant pudding. While I most certainly push for a diet that is as natural as possible, occasionally we need to rely on the miracles of science to aid us in our journey. In other words, there are some scientifically created chemicals in this product. That being said, it is extremely inexpensive, versatile, comes in many flavors, and most importantly, is very low in calories. Just one example of what you can do with sugar free instant pudding is 35 calorie pudding pops. Inexpensive Popsicle molds can be found at most supermarkets. Simply prepare a box of pudding and pour it into the mold. You can also beat 2 cups of sugar free whipped topping into chilled pudding to make a fantastic low calorie mousse. This is another great way to let your creative spirit take over. The possibilities of this product are almost endless. Imagine 35 calorie pudding pops! Go ahead and have two.

One of the problems that I have with most of the diets and programs out there is the inclusion of a "cheat" day. I have never been able to get my mind around a concept that expects an individual to adhere to a rather strict diet for 6 days yet on the 7th day permits the individual to eat whatever they wish and blow the week's progress. I believe this to be a major step in the wrong direction. You must understand that you can still have an occasional treat. Rewarding yourself can be a wonderful and very positive experience. The key to this process is a shift in your thinking and a general lifestyle change. Consistency is at the heart of the process. If you eat the right foods in the right daily proportions, and are getting proper exercise than an occasional 350 calorie brownie will not become a major setback. It is also important not to allow that occasional treat to cause you to feel guilt. This is a negative emotion of your own creation. If you begin to feel guilty just remember that you have already consumed the treat. That event is now in the past. You must set that aside and move forward. Just remember that a treat is just that. It is the exception and not the rule. It's something that happens infrequently. Let's say that you go to a party and really go crazy. You eat and drink everything in sight. The next day you are angry and upset that you just assassinated your diet. Your mind can go into a kind of panic mode and you begin to think, "I've done it now...all of that hard work was for nothing". You are thinking this way because you have literally created that negative emotion that is leading you in the wrong direction. You went out and pigged out one night. So what? Most likely, you didn't consume anything that will cause you to gain 10 pounds in an evening. Feeling badly about one night's indiscretion is the wrong way of thinking. Instead of dwelling on what you consumed that evening, focus on the good time that you had while doing it. Simply get up the next morning, smile, look for one of your signs, and go about your meal and exercise routine as usual. Ladies, never feel bad about having a good time. That is what life is all about.

On the subject of having a good time, one of the questions that inevitably comes up as a fitness instructor is well, alcohol consumption. We as adults are aware of the risks of alcohol consumption whether they are physical, legal, emotional, etc. The truth is that alcohol is one of those guilty pleasures that we indulge in even though we know that it is not good for us. Alcohol is also a known depressant. I would be thrilled if you didn't consume any alcohol during this process; however if you are over 21 then let's be realistic. Red wine is said to have powerful antioxidant properties and other health benefits. The only problem with red wine is that it can be in the neighborhood of 250 calories per serving. So basically, one 8oz glass of red wine can be compared to the calories in your favorite chocolate bar. We have to be mindful of our calories and unfortunately alcohol is usually not calorie friendly; however there are a few exceptions. White rum is 65 calories per ounce and has 0 carbs. So in theory, a person could have say 3 rum and diet sodas and still only be around 195 calories. By comparison, 3 rum and diet sodas have roughly 75% fewer calories than 3 glasses of red wine. Beers are usually high in calories and carbohydrates; however there are a few lower calorie, lower carb options available. If beer happens to be your drink of choice then I would certainly recommend going with one of those options. Just remember that lower carb beer means lower carbs than regular beer and not necessarily low in carbs. You will want to avoid bourbon as well as most liqueurs as they tend to be higher in both calories and carbs. If you chose to consume alcohol then do so in extreme moderation and of course never ever drink and drive.

Another very important part of your journey is shopping. The supermarket can be one of the most important parts of your success. It can also be a place to make some serious mistakes that can send you down the wrong path. The trick is to know how to shop properly. There is most certainly a right, and a wrong way to shop for meals. I'm sure that you have heard the old saying about never shopping hungry. That is actually a very true statement. When you are hungry and in the midst of all that food it is very easy to make some pretty bad choices. Your mind is overwhelmed by all of the available options and that makes something as easy as a box of snack cakes look pretty good. You can also go into the supermarket with the best of intentions and make mistakes that can hinder your progress by simply being unprepared. The best way to approach shopping day is to make it just that, pick one set day of the week and make an appointment with yourself and stick to it. It can be any time day or night; however I have always had the best results with shopping right after a meal. The theory being that you are already full so hunger will be much less of a factor in your mind. Make a plan. Plan your meals out on a weekly basis. Use your smartphone, laptop, or even a notebook and write out everything that you are going to consume for the week. You will want to create a basic itemized list and it is crucial that you have it with you on shopping day. You should, if at all possible be prepared to purchase everything that you are going to consume for the entire week in one shopping trip. This may not always be practical; however think of it this way, the more you expose yourself to the foods that you are trying to avoid, the more likely you are to have a misstep. So it is very important to go in armed with your list and to be very efficient while in the supermarket. Become a supermarket ninja. Your shopping list should be followed to the letter. Don't walk the entire store as again, you will be walking past some pretty serious temptation. Make your shopping trip as much of a surgical, in and out procedure as possible. This is not a good time to stop and smell the roses especially if you are at the beginning of your journey. Another fantastic tip and I cannot take credit for this one as it was provided by a client of mine, is to use your smartphone and take some photos of your signs. That way you can always refer to your signs when you are mobile and need to focus.

Let's talk about treats or weekly rewards. Rewarding yourself from time to time is a good thing. A treat at the right time can be just thing to bend, but not break your weekly routine. The trick is not to allow one small indiscretion to lead to feelings of guilt or a domino effect. That is why I do not recommend treats that are outside of your plan for at least the first several weeks. A treat should be a celebration of your work and progress. Think of it as the pop of the champagne cork. When you feel that the time is right, and you are ready for something really special, then it is time for our next exercise. This can work with many different kinds of naughty foods; however I have found that this works best with pastry and or baked goods. On your shopping trip, take a moment to stop by the bakery counter. Look in that case and really take it all in. Pick out one item that looks really good. Go ahead and make it something that is sinfully rich. Don't worry about the calorie math as this is a reward for doing such an amazing job to get to this point in the process. Again, this should only be attempted several weeks into your journey. Try to select a piece of thick frosted cake or perhaps a really gooey brownie. Go ahead and have the baker wrap up your selection and finish your shopping trip. When you arrive home, I would like for you to place your reward directly into the freezer. No nibbles, no samples, no peeking, and you thought you were going to eat it didn't you? :) Let your treat freeze as solid as possible. Now let's set a date to enjoy your reward. Think of it as a personal party. It could be tomorrow or several days from now. Now that you have a date set, try and put the treat out of your mind and go on with your regular routine. The idea is to have this delightful treat within your reach; however you must take the time to allow it to thaw before consuming it. Think of it as a "cooling off" period. We are freezing this treat because in its frozen form it cannot be easily consumed at the spur of the moment. You cannot have a bad experience and use it for immediate comfort food. Remember that it is a reward, not a Valium, and should be consumed at the right time and for the right reasons.

Now that we have discussed how to shop and what to shop for, let's discuss where to shop. When it comes to shopping, your choice of supermarket and shopping technique can greatly affect your budget. Everyone enjoys saving money. Getting a good deal on something always makes you feel great. If you think about it, it really is a great time in history to be a bargain shopper. Look at all of the deals that find their way to your mailbox on a weekly basis. There are many fantastic coupon sites on the internet that can really help you save money. Over the years, I have become a big fan of members only warehouse shopping. I have found that in most cases, I can purchase double the amount of meat from a warehouse for roughly the same cost as what I would be spending at my local supermarket. Most member only warehouse clubs charge an annual fee; however I have found that minimal cost to be well worth it in what I save on meats and other bulk items. Go check some of these places out. I am also a huge fan of coupons. In today's world, if you want a discount or deal on something, it is very easy to go online and find a coupon or discount on just about anything that you wish to shop for. It really does add up.

There are also weight loss programs that basically create a meal plan for you and ship the food directly to your home. While I do believe that some of these programs are worthwhile, I could never really get my mind around having my food shipped to my home in the mail. I have also had the opportunity to check some of the ingredients. Many of these products have chemicals and preservatives that I honestly wouldn't feed to my pet. Again, some of these programs do have some pretty decent food offerings and support systems if you are fortunate enough to be able to afford them. Remember to always keep it simple. Simply put, the more simplified your dietary process becomes, the greater your chances of success will be.

Let's discuss some of the many temptations that you will have to overcome during your personal journey. Your journey will have some obstacles along the way and you will hit some of them. The trick is in how you deal with these obstacles. Let's face it, in today's society it is nearly impossible to avoid being bombarded by food advertisements. They pop up everywhere from television to signs on a local bus. This level of temptation can certainly be a distraction to the untrained mind. One of my biggest distractions has always been late night restaurant television commercials. They just make everything look so good. This can be an unavoidable obstacle; however I adopted a method to combat these late night food trolls. When you are enjoying your favorite television program and a tempting advertisement slithers its way onto your screen simply change the channel for a few minutes. You can always hit the power button and wait it out. The good news is that as you move along this journey your mind will naturally become much more disciplined and everyday temptations like the aforementioned really will become much less of a distraction.

Another one of the things that many people struggle with at first is a very basic human instinct. I'm speaking of the hand-to-mouth instinct. Those of us that have been overeaters in the past know exactly what I'm speaking of. It is the tendency to constantly snack and basically put something into our mouths. This can be a difficult habit to break especially at first. Luckily you have many options at your disposal. Sugarless gum can be a very positive tool for these types of situations. Another great asset is sugarless hard candies. There are many varieties of sugarless gum, mints, and candies available and most add very few calories to your daily intake. Some of my favorites are around ten calories each. Remember that even though these products really do help to scratch that itch, they too must be consumed in moderation.

Chapter 3

The She Time Body

ow that we have discussed the proper diet and mindset, it is time to get to the next and final leg of your journey. I am speaking of your body. Specifically, I am speaking of your current metabolic rate. We have all heard the theory that an object at rest tends to stay and rest, and an object in motion tends to stay in motion, right? That is truly a correct statement. When the body is stationary for long periods of time it basically goes into a stand-by mode. In other words, your metabolism decreases and therefore the body requires much less caloric intake to function. The problem is that when your metabolic rate tanks, you are still consuming just as many calories as you would if you were an active person, or a person with a higher metabolism. The key to weight loss in my humble opinion really is your metabolic rate. Now that we are eating and thinking correctly it is time to take the next step. The truth is that your new diet is basically designed to raise your metabolic rate naturally. Now you are empowering your body to do exactly what it was designed to do. You have drastically cut your caloric intake, you have been drinking green tea and you have no doubt begun to feel the difference in your clothing at this point. Now to really kick things into overdrive, it's time to get up and get moving. It's She Time ladies.

Honestly, this is a challenging chapter to create because there are so many wonderful fitness options available. There are fitness DVDs, gym memberships, group fitness classes, yoga, and the list goes on. How many of us have purchased exercise equipment for our home that is now sitting in our bedroom playing the part of clothing rack or plant hanger? Remember that there are three basic rules to exercise: stretch out before beginning any activity, start slowly, and go at your own pace. As we are all different people with different lifestyles and needs, I will start with the basics of movement and move forward to more challenging aspects of fitness such as group fitness classes. Again ladies, it is extremely important to consult your physician before starting any exercise program. Always remember to start slowly and move forward at your own pace. Your journey is not a race and it isn't supposed to be. It will take some time but that is ok because as we all know the finer things in life take time. That is what makes them the finer things.

Let's talk a bit more about weight gain. You must remember that weight gain is not about who you are. It is about who you were. Fat takes time to manifest and grow. It does not magically appear overnight. Weight gain is literally a product of your past that is affecting your current reality. You are currently in the process of changing your reality. You have already begun the process of changing your personal negatives into positives. Your bathroom scale seems like a nice item to have in your home and it actually is. The scale however can also be a fairly serious obstacle during your journey. In fact, when not used properly, it has the potential to be a major bump in the road. One of the first things that many of my new fitness clients want to do is to hit the scale. They do this because they want to know their exact weight, and they want to hear it from a professional. You will need to know your weight because that is the starting point of your journey. The problem with the bathroom scale is that women tend to want to weigh themselves far too often. To many, it almost becomes an obsession. What you must understand about the female body is that there are many factors that can cause you to gain small amounts of weight naturally and rapidly. As an example, it is not uncommon for a woman to gain several pounds right before a menstrual cycle. I have seen this upset many over the years. This is the reason that weighing too often can cause you to feel stress and lose your focus. That is another major step in the wrong direction. Your clothing is actually the best way to realize your progress. When your clothing becomes loose, and this happens faster than you might think, then that is real, tangible progress. That is your reason to celebrate. You must capture those feelings and emotions and refer to them often. Good feelings of progress always bring about even more progress. Remember to feel gratitude toward yourself because it is you who are making this new reality manifest. Pat yourself on the back. Make some She Time.

Let's talk about fat. There are many misconceptions about fat in terms of what it is and how to lose it. I could go into several medical and scientific descriptions; however I don't want to bore you. Let's think of fat as simply stored energy that is waiting to be used. One of the most popular questions that I have had over the years is about targeted weight loss. Women will ask about the best ways to lose say belly fat, perhaps arm fat, could be rear fat, you get the idea. They are looking for targeted weight loss. Think of how many belly whacker devices that you have seen advertised on television. You know the old story; the model has belly fat, starts using the whacker and presto, amazing six-pack right? Unfortunately, fat does not work that way. The reality is that there is no such thing as targeted weight loss.

The entire body must lose weight as a whole. My experience has been that most women tend to lose their newest fat first. In other words, they lose the latest fat that their body has created, and then they lose older fat and so on. I think of fat like an onion. You lose one layer, then another, then another, and so on. While I am an incredibly big believer in the theory that any and all exercise is good, some of these products and their descriptions are misleading at best.

While we are on the subject of fat, let's discuss what I like to call the plateau effect. People that have a great deal of weight to lose tend to drop a great deal at first, then after several weeks their weight loss either significantly slows or stops for a period of time. This is the plateau effect. This happens to both male and female bodies; however the bad news is that in my experience, it tends to last longer in women. This can be very discouraging because it will happen even though you are doing all of the right things. You must understand that this is a natural process and it does in fact happen to everyone. Remember that this is a temporary situation. The trick here is to anticipate this bump in the road and not to allow it to change your thought process. This effect can last several weeks so it is extremely important to roll with it. This is another reason why I always push my clients to leave the scale alone. After a few weeks your body will begin to lose weight at a faster rate again and you will feel as though you are right back in the game.

It is very important that you understand that the weight loss journey is not about speed, it is about consistency. You are in this for the long haul and you will get to your destination as long as you believe deep down that you are making progress. Remember, forward thinking is always a step in the right direction. You have a program, you have a mission, and you have a plan. Stay on the path and don't allow anything to corrupt your positive mindset. The plateau effect can and will be a tough time and honestly, this is where many women give up. Again, it is very important to remember that this is a temporary situation.

At this point in your journey you have begun to master your thoughts and emotions. You are also beginning to understand why positive thoughts throughout this process are the key to success. You are no doubt becoming aware that positive thoughts really do become positive things because you are seeing this in nearly every aspect of your life. That is a wonderful thing. Your personal reality really is beginning to change for the better and the best part about it is that you are making it happen.

Our next goal is to begin to stimulate your metabolism and learn ways to keep it accelerated on a permanent basis. The best thing that you can do to begin this process is to simply get moving. A sedentary lifestyle is the absolute worst thing for your metabolism. Many of us become sedentary for a number of different reasons. Being sedentary may seem like a tough habit to break but the good news is that once you break that pattern, it becomes easier to stay in motion on a regular basis. It's time to get that heart pumping. I am certainly not suggesting going right to the half marathon, I am talking about starting slow and steady. To some people this may seem a little intimidating but the truth is you need to begin to get physical. It is time to empower your body. You are about to gradually turn your body into the efficient machine that it is designed to be. There are infinite ways to get in motion and the good news is that most of them are easy and free. What I am about to explain is very important and if this method is followed properly, it will greatly accelerate your weight loss. You will also begin to feel even better physically in a very short time.

I say this from personal experience, I say this from observing my clients, the absolute best thing that you can do to stimulate your metabolism is to wake up in the morning and get moving. I am talking about up, to the bathroom, and then get moving in that order. The idea behind early morning exercise is fairly simple, when you jumpstart your metabolism first thing in the morning the body will tend to maintain a higher metabolic rate throughout your day. In other words, your body will burn more calories while at rest throughout the day because of your morning exercise. This is when you will start noticing significant changes to your body. This is the point at which you start shopping for a smaller size.

Let's try another exercise. Tomorrow morning when you wake up it is time to make a few minutes of She Time. I want you to stand up with your feet close together. Just try to find a natural stance, and hold both of your arms straight down to your sides with your palms flat. Take five very deep breaths. Clear your mind of any thoughts other than your breath and think of the lemon or whatever object you may have replaced it with. Now completely exhale and in one deep breath bring your arms straight out to the side and above your head. Your arms should be moving in one fluid motion. Now exhale as you bring your arms back down to a resting position and repeat. It is very important to clear your mind during this exercise. You should give yourself at least five minutes with this. This exercise will help to center your mind and to prepare your body for the day. You must remember that exercise must never be viewed as a chore. That is a step in the wrong direction. Every workout becomes a victory the moment that you start it.

As much as your diet is the fuel for the vehicle during your journey, exercise is the actual vehicle that will take you there. Your exercise routine is the last part of the puzzle. We call it a routine because it is just that, it is something that must be done on a regular basis. A great way to get in motion is by simply walking. Get up in the morning and take a fifteen minute walk. Walk around your neighborhood, take a stroll around your complex, you can even hit your treadmill if you happen to own one. Walking is a very good, low impact way to get some exercise and to get your metabolism started. You don't have to walk very far at first. Test your current limit and then set a further goal for next time. Feel free to change it up with more challenging terrain. Walking really is a fantastic way to start your day. You should walk everywhere you can. Walking is also a wonderful lunchtime activity. Taking the stairs is another fantastic way to get some exercise. Forget about the elevator and take the stairs. If you have ever had the opportunity to watch many female track and field athletes train, one of the things that you are likely to see is stair training. I mean just look at their thighs and calves. Working the stairs is amazing for your cardio, legs, and especially rear. Again, this is not a race so it is very important to take things slowly. Feel free to put in some earbuds. Music is a great motivator and can promote good feelings and mood. The right music can bring back positive thoughts and memories. Those thoughts and emotions are exactly what you want to be holding in your mind. So feel free to use your new power of visualization and take a trip down memory lane.

Getting yourself in motion can be a challenge. For many, it may be a new experience. What you must understand is that your daily exercise routine only gets easier the more you do it. As it becomes easier, you will begin to realize that easier means positive progress. When it becomes too easy then you know it is time to up your game. Your body will literally dictate your pace once you begin to master it. Let's think about old photos of people. I am speaking of Old West photos, or could be turn of the 20th century photos. You should look some of these up. You won't see a great many overweight people in them. The reason is fairly simple; they were always in motion and didn't eat crap. Now don't get me wrong, most folks back in "them" days didn't exactly eat right. Frankly, they didn't know how to eat right. They just had far fewer choices of said crap than we have today. Keep in mind that motion is your very best friend at this point. An object in motion tends to stay in motion. You need to keep reminding yourself of that. Believe it, believe it, believe it. You have set out to empower your body, and you will empower your body. You need to own the thoughts of forward progress because progress is becoming your new reality.

It has been proven scientifically that exercise and motion stimulate the release of endorphins from the brain that make you feel absolutely amazing. I am sure that you have heard of the term "runner's high" right? Well it is a very real thing and endorphins make that possible. It has been said that some people even get addicted to that high. I have a neighbor that will jog in a foot of snow. Your body really does want to work with your mind and when they come together, you feel great. It is a gift from Mother Nature. It is a reward for doing the right things. Honestly, when I work out in the morning I find that I am in a much better mood all day. Try it and I am sure that you will agree. I simply cannot stress enough the importance of motion and consistency. Seriously, first thing in the morning is the way to go. Now it is time to get up and get moving.

People that have a good deal of extra weight tend to begin to lose it fairly rapidly with a change of diet and lifestyle. The body really does not want to carry around all of that extra energy. It forces every system in the body to work much harder than it was designed to do. This is why overweight people have a host of health issues. Being overweight puts you at risk of heart attack, diabetes, and several other debilitating conditions. Your ankle, knee, hip joints aren't happy either. So the body really will work to eliminate that extra energy if given the chance. I have personally worked with people who were diabetic while overweight, and no longer diabetic after a major weight loss. Your DNA has a blueprint of basically how your body is supposed to be. When we add a large amount of additional mass in the form of fat to the equation, the body's systems simply cannot keep up. When this happens, the only choice that we have is to compensate with medications.

One of the stories that I share with my clients is about my grandmother. My grandparents were of the World War II generation that lacked the dietary sciences that we enjoy today. At around age 60, my grandmother began to have multiple health issues. These issues were brought on for the most part, by a lifetime of improper diet and exercise. So for the last 25 years of her life my grandmother was forced to extend her life by taking several different kinds of medications, several times a day. I can still see it in my mind today, a wicker basket full of pill bottles on the kitchen table. Hey, they had to be taken with food. No matter where she would go her medications had to follow. The bottom line is that being chained to medications prevented her from living out her golden years to the fullest in many ways. Years of smoking and her oxygen tank certainly didn't help for that matter but more on smoking later. There are so many reasons to stay off of medications that the reasons could be a book by themselves. While I both realize and agree that there is most certainly a place for drugs and medicines in our society, I prefer to stay healthy and not need them. Let's think about being dependent on medication for the rest of your life. Drugs are expensive and almost always lead to side effects, some of which can be very serious. The next time that you see a drug advertisement on television, look at the fine print. Just look at all of the possible side effects from taking many of these medications. Imagine what would happen if you were taking one of these medications long-term and for whatever reason the medications were no longer available. Best bet is to keep your body working the way in which it was intended and to avoid the need for medications all together. If you are already suffering from a medical condition, you might be hard pressed to find a medical professional that doesn't agree that weight loss will go a long way toward treatment and recovery. Let's rock that metabolism!

Now that you have been in motion for some time I am certain that you are physically feeling a difference. You will notice that you suddenly have a great deal more energy. You are most likely sleeping less. This is because your metabolic rate has improved a great deal simply by adopting the habit of getting up and getting in motion. After a few short weeks, you will no doubt be ready to up your game and get even more active. Always remember that activity leads to even more activity. Not only does activity lead to a healthier lifestyle, it actually tends to become a lifestyle of its own. This is where your personal reality begins to change even further into positive territory. You are on the right path because you have the right formula. Some might say that it is really just as simple as proper diet and exercise and I certainly would not argue that point. I would however remind you that your mind and thought process is just as important. Focus creates strength, strength creates resolve, and resolve creates a new reality. Thoughts really do become reality whether they are positive or negative, so it is important to use all of your tools to stay in a positive mindset.

Let's make some She Time and try another exercise. Now that you have been in constant motion for a while it is time to take you exercise routine to the next level. Get up in the morning and start with the breathing technique that you learned earlier in this chapter. Now it's time to have some fun. I would like for you to put on some music and dance. That's right, I said dance. Find a nice private area, crank your favorite tunes and literally get funky. Listen to the music and let your body naturally move to the beat. Don't concern yourself with any particular step or motion. It honestly doesn't even have to be pretty. Remember that there are no cameras, no reality television judges, and nobody is watching so feel free to just let yourself go. You would honestly be surprised at how much exercise you can get from doing a simple dance like the twist. Enjoy this because it really is a fun activity. Use the power of visualization and put yourself in that ballroom. Go out to that nightclub. Shake it girl, this moment is all about you. Always remember to start slowly.

Just getting your feet moving and allowing your body to sway is fantastic exercise. You are at the point at which your daily exercise should be causing your heart to beat at a faster rate and if you can feel that, it means that your body is in the zone. You are literally feeling your metabolic rate increase. It means that you are burning calories and that is exactly where you need to be. Of course you will begin to feel those endorphins kick in and that feels wonderful. Another thing to remember is that when you really get moving it can cause minor muscle soreness. This is natural and every person that goes from a sedentary state to one of consistent motion must deal with it. Muscle soreness is a temporary condition and should only last for a few days. Most people would probably say that the third day of muscle soreness is the worst and I would tend to agree. Just remember that minor soreness is part of the journey and at the risk of being cliché once again, no pain no gain. You should think of temporary, minor soreness as progress. Revel in that progress as it really does mean improvement, and that is a positive change in your personal reality. It is very important not to allow minor pain to change your routine or your thoughts. Of course, if you find yourself in terrible pain then stop what you are doing and seek medical attention but otherwise just understand that minor aches and pains are part of the journey. This is a temporary condition. Push through it. We have a term for exercise that we feel for a few hours afterward, we call that a workout ladies. Now you are more than just in motion, you are on the move.

As valuable as getting in motion has become for your metabolism, at some point you will be ready to up your game and try something more advanced. There are so many options available to you in the modern world. You can choose anything from classes on DVD, a gym membership, cycling, yoga, and many other options. I will cover a few of the more popular options; however it is important to remember to get into a routine of what makes you the most comfortable. It is also extremely important to remember that whichever method, or combination of methods you choose, it must never be viewed as a chore. It is just another step in the journey to success.

Let's discuss yoga. The simple Wiki definition of yoga is as follows; Yoga is an ancient discipline from India. Yoga uses breathing techniques, posture exercise and meditation to center the mind and body. The actual definition is somewhat more complex. Yoga is as much a spiritual experience as it is an exercise. It really is a great fit for your particular program. Many yoga practitioners claim that the practice opens up new and different parts of the mind and through that process, a higher level of consciousness and state of awareness is born. Honestly, yoga may indeed be one of the best ways to get started in a group fitness environment. Yoga will also work muscles that you probably didn't know you had. Though many yoga disciplines may not be as much of a heart pumping exercise per se, it tends to make up for some of that with muscle toning postures and movements that may be just what the doctor ordered for someone beginning her fitness journey.

Yoga really does help a person get the mind into a positive state and ladies that is precisely where we want to be at this point of the journey. Another great thing about yoga is that anyone can do it. Classes are abundant, affordable, and are available for any skill level. One thing that those of you that are new to group fitness may appreciate about yoga classes is the fact that they are low impact and generally held in a very non-threatening environment. The yoga subject is much too vast and complex to explain here; however there are hundreds, if not thousands of videos and publications that you can view for more in depth info. Personally, I would simply suggest that you pick up a yoga mat, find a class, find a buddy, and just jump right in. Always remember that fortune favors the bold.

Let's discuss fitness centers and what they can do for you. Before we proceed any further I want to clear up some common misconceptions about fitness centers. The first thing that you should know is that absolutely nobody is looking at you. Honestly, most people do not join a fitness center to people watch and most neighborhood fitness centers are not "pickup" spots. Everyone else that is sharing that space with you is in their own little world and that is a promise. The next common gym misconception is that if you use weights your body will become too muscular and that you can She Hulk out. I promise that this is not going to happen with any kind of a reasonable workout. You must understand that female bodybuilders workout 4-6 hours per day, every day. They are also on a much stricter and frankly, radical diet than anything that we are discussing here. I know this because I have worked with clients that were actually striving for the She Hulk thing. We got it done but it honestly wasn't easy. This is nothing to worry about.

Sadly, statistically speaking, about half of the people that purchase fitness center memberships stop attending after the first few visits. The reason why is very simple and at the risk of sounding unkind, they simply have no idea what they are doing. They go in and get started without any knowledge or supervision and the next day they cannot get out of bed from the pain and soreness. It's akin to laying your hand on something hot and getting burned. Once your hand is burned, your natural instinct is to not do that thing that caused you pain again. Our body senses pain to basically keep us alive and in one piece. It is imperative that you avoid this very common gym mistake. Creating that kind of pain for yourself is most definitely a step in the wrong direction.

The best way to avoid this is to first take everything slowly and second, find a gym that offers a few free personal training sessions. Now I will be honest with you, the free sessions are designed to get you to purchase more sessions. If you are able to afford a trainer then that is fantastic otherwise you will want to get the most out of those free sessions that the fitness center offers. My advice is to insist that your trainer create a beginning program for you. Get them to create a workout chart for you based on what you wish to accomplish. Don't be afraid to ask lots of questions. They are there to assist you. If you are planning on hiring a trainer then you should ask for multiple references. Actually contact those references and ask questions. If this person is a good trainer, then his/her references will be thrilled to speak with you. If a trainer only has one or two references to share then you are probably going to be speaking to the trainer's Aunt Martha so be selective about who you hire and why.

To be honest, I believe in my heart of hearts that purchasing a gym membership is the way to go. A gym membership is fantastic for a host of different reasons not the least of which is the fact that many have everything that you would need under one roof. Most medium to large fitness centers offer amenities such as weights, resistance equipment, a variety of group fitness classes, cardio equipment, personal training, and some even offer massage therapy. All of that for an affordable monthly fee. All you have to do is take that step. Visit your local fitness center and take the tour. The experience may be a bit overwhelming to some at first; however I promise that you will get over that after the second visit.

Let's discuss the buddy system of support. Having a workout and dieting partner can be a wonderful motivational asset. Most people tend to get much more out of their exercise experience by sharing it with someone else. It is always nice to have a partner to pick you up and offer support when you need it; however you must have basic compatibility. In other words, you should share very similar fitness goals and have a compatible schedule. You need to understand that while a trusty workout buddy can be a big help it is incredibly important to have your own personal program. This journey is about you and you alone. I have personally witnessed situations where lady workout partners were doing very well together and then suddenly one of them would stop working out for whatever reason. The remaining workout partner would stop shortly thereafter. It is important not to fall into this very common trap. Again this is your personal She Time and though you may decide to share it, you really need to believe in your heart of hearts that this is all about you. Always be prepared to go it alone.

Let's discuss my personal favorite fitness activity. I'm speaking of group fitness classes. I taught a class of my own development for many years and I can tell you that it's effective because it is so much fun. It's almost as if the entire room becomes one team, one body. The energy is incredible. There are so many different group fitness classes to choose from. You should try several different classes until you find the one that is right for you. Many group fitness classes are a serious workout that you will be feeling for hours after you leave. You will also enjoy that runner's high that I mentioned earlier. It really does become addictive and that is a great thing considering a good class can burn several hundred calories in an hour. The instructor of a group fitness class is usually a very interesting person. They aren't there for the money as it really isn't worth mentioning. Those instructors are there because they have a calling. They are there simply to help you achieve your fitness goals period. Group classes may seem difficult and even intimidating at first; however after you get a few classes under your belt, you will begin to see yourself picking up the pace and matching the rest of the class. I have personally watched ladies transform from huff and puff to great cardio condition in my own classes over the years, and it happens faster than you think. Class is also an outstanding place to make friends and perhaps even meet a good workout buddy. You can do this. You will do this. You have all of the tools that you need to advance to the next level so hit the gas and let's get going!

We have just covered some of, in my opinion, the best fitness options and final component of your journey. The truth is that everyone is different which means that everyone's life situation is different. You may not be able afford a fitness center membership. You may not be able to afford a personal trainer. You may prefer not to be part of the public eye and that is just fine. You can still absolutely afford some She Time. You deserve it. Someone in your life may need to deal with the fact that you need She Time. They will get over it, I promise. If the public eye is not your thing then there are several other options available for you to get your sweat on. There are classes on the internet and DVDs that you can participate in right in your own living room. Cycling and rollerblading are also fantastic options to get that metabolism cranked into high gear. Again the key to any successful weight loss program is consistency. Find an exercise activity that you enjoy and make it a routine. One of the most common questions that I get asked when someone is starting their journey is How often should I exercise? The answer is dependent on many factors but the easy answer is at least three to five times a week. The truth of the matter is that when it comes to an exercise routine, you get as much out of it as you put into it. Simply put, the more that you exercise the higher your metabolic rate rises and the more weight your body will lose. Again the key is consistency. Your exercise routine should be just that a routine. You should be doing it at least three times per week. If you have a good deal of weight to lose then I would suggest hitting your routine even more often. Remember that to get the best results from your program, you really should exercise first thing in the morning. It really does help.

I would like to take a minute to discuss a taboo subject in the fitness world. I am speaking of cigarette smoking. Ladies I will be honest with you. I was a smoking athlete. I remember sneaking off behind the gym to have one last smoke before class and would pray that nobody would see me. Nicotine is an incredibly addictive drug. Cigarettes are expensive, nasty, and they will eventually kill you. Honestly, I am still addicted to nicotine; however I discovered something that changed my life. I am speaking of electronic cigarettes. Ladies these things work. They are inexpensive, easy to use, come in multiple flavors and nicotine levels, and can be found at any e-cig shop. If you do smoke then you really should consider trying an e-cig. It may take a few days to get used to them over regular cigarettes; however when you do, you will feel a major difference in your health and fitness almost immediately. I also did not suffer the usual weight gain from quitting smoking by switching to the e-cig. Do yourself a favor if you and smoke stop into an e-cig shop and try one.

In closing I would just like to remind you that you already have everything you need for your journey. It is important to remember that any fitness journey must start in the mind and extend to the body. You have purchased this book because you are ready to change your life for the better. This is not a race and significant weight loss does take time and effort; however when you start dropping dress sizes you will become very proud of yourself and you should be. Weight loss really is a life changing event. You will be pleasantly surprised by the reactions of the people who are close to you be they family members, coworkers, and even your doctor. You will be much more productive in life because putting it simply; you will be healthy and happier. Basically you are turning your body from a dumpster into the efficient machine that it was created to be and the best part about it is that you are doing this for yourself. This is a gift of life for you from yourself. The only thing that you need to do at this point is to set a date and start your program. Just remember that She Time is your time and if necessary, you may need to make others work around you. This is one of the most important things you can do for yourself and you are about to make it happen. Be happy, be positive, be fit, be safe, and claim your She Time. Congratulations you are about to become the next fitness success.

9 781973 288930